LOW-SUGAR

FOOD LIST

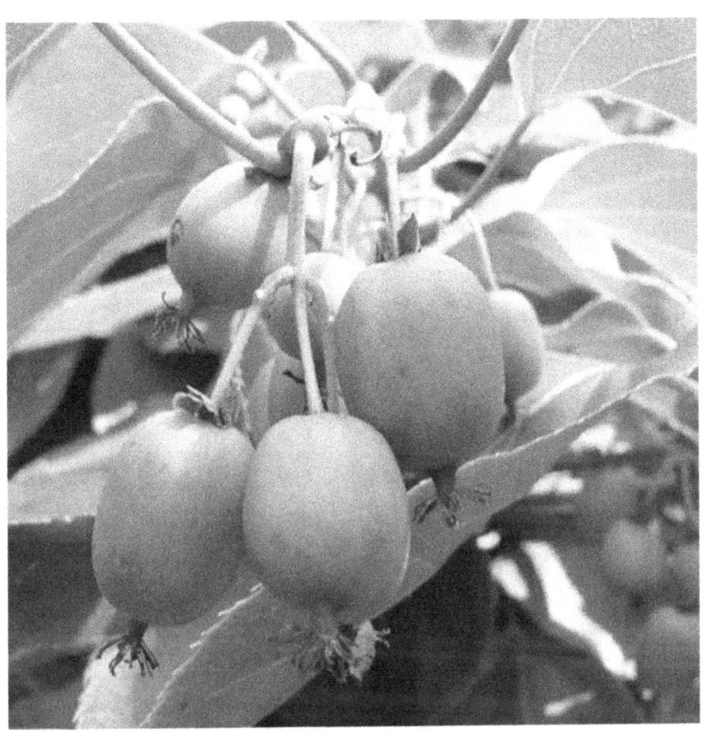

LORENE PEACHEY

DISCLAIMER

The content within this book reflects my thoughts, experiences, and beliefs. It is meant for informational and entertainment purposes. While I have taken great care to provide accurate information, I cannot guarantee the absolute correctness or applicability of the content to every individual or situation. Please consult with relevant professionals for advice specific to your needs.

TO GAIN ACCESS TO MORE BOOK BY THE AUTHOR SCAN THE QR CODE

TABLE OF CONTENTS

INTRODUCTION

In the labyrinth of life's nutritional maze, I am Nutrionist Lorene Peachey, a devoted explorer who has dedicated countless years to unraveling the secrets of healthy living. My journey began not as a mere academic pursuit but as a personal odyssey rooted in a desire to redefine the way we nourish our bodies. Welcome to the realm of low-sugar culinary delights, a testament to my undying passion for crafting recipes that not only tantalize the taste buds but also elevate well-being.

As I tread through the corridors of nutritional wisdom, my heart echoes with the joy of discovery. Picture a vibrant kitchen, filled with the aroma of fresh ingredients and the sizzle of a pan, as I embarked on a quest to demystify the enigma of low-sugar living. This is not just a journey; it's a labor of love that has spanned a quarter of a century, a symphony of flavors orchestrated with the precision of a seasoned conductor.

What motivated me to dedicate my life to this culinary exploration? It wasn't just the pursuit of professional expertise; it was a deeply personal revelation. I, like many of you, have danced with the highs and lows of life's culinary temptations. There were times when sugary confections whispered sweet promises, only to leave me grappling with the consequences of indulgence.

Have you ever questioned the impact of your dietary choices on your health and happiness? Have you pondered the potential dangers lurking in the shadows of high-sugar lifestyles? The truth is, our bodies are intricate canvases, and every morsel we consume paints a picture of our well-being. I found myself at a crossroads, facing the undeniable truth that what we eat shapes not only our physical health but also our emotional resilience.

Now, let's delve into the profound questions that stir the very essence of our being: What if I told you that the journey to a healthier, happier you begins with the choices you make in your kitchen? What if the secret to vitality lies in the art of savoring flavors that dance on your palate without compromising your well-being? These are the questions that set the stage for a transformative odyssey, a journey I invite you to embark upon with me.

The dangers of excessive sugar consumption are well-documented, casting a shadow on our health and vitality. It's not just about the visible consequences – the extra pounds and the occasional energy crashes. It's about the silent havoc sugar wreaks on our internal systems, from elevating the risk of chronic diseases to playing havoc with our mental well-being. Picture the momentary joy of indulging in a sugary treat, only to be followed by the crash that leaves you feeling drained and defeated. Is that the life we envision for ourselves?

Enter the realm of low-sugar living, where the benefits extend far beyond the physical. Picture a life where your energy levels soar, your mood stabilizes, and your mind becomes a beacon of clarity. Imagine waking up in the morning with a sense of vitality that propels you through the day, unburdened by the sluggishness that often accompanies high-sugar diets. The advantages are not just about shedding pounds; they're about embracing a lifestyle that empowers you to live your best life.

This book is not a mere compilation of recipes; it's a lifeline extended to those who seek to break free from the shackles of unhealthy eating. It's a companion on your journey to rediscovering the joy of food – a joy that extends beyond mere sustenance to become a celebration of life itself.

In the chapters that follow, you will find a curated collection of recipes that bear the fruits of my years of research and experience. These are not just dishes; they are a testament to the art of nourishing the body and soul. Each recipe is a brushstroke on the canvas of well-being, crafted with love and purpose to bring joy to your dining table.

But this book is not just about me; it's about the countless lives that have been touched by the magic of low-sugar living. Picture a community of individuals who have embraced this lifestyle and witnessed the transformative power of their choices. The stories are inspiring – tales of weight loss, renewed energy, and a renewed zest for life. As you flip through these pages, you are not alone; you become a part of a movement that celebrates the joy of mindful eating.

What sets this book apart is not just the sumptuous recipes; it's the underlying philosophy that resonates with the very fabric of our humanity. It's an invitation to savor life in all its richness without compromising our health. It's a call to action, urging you to reclaim your well-being, one delicious bite at a time.

The journey we are about to embark upon is not a rigid dietary plan; it's a flexible, adaptable approach to nourishment. It's about fostering a relationship with food that is built on mindfulness, moderation, and a celebration of the bountiful flavors nature has to offer. As we navigate the culinary landscapes together, remember that this is not a restrictive diet; it's a culinary adventure that invites you to savor the diverse tapestry of low-sugar living.

So, fasten your seatbelts, my dear readers, for we are about to embark on a journey that transcends the boundaries of conventional cookbooks. This is not just a book; it's a manifesto for a life well-lived, a symphony of flavors that will resonate with your taste buds and nourish your soul. Let the adventure begin.

Contact the Author

Thank you for reading my book! I would love to hear from you, whether you have feedback, questions, or just want to share your thoughts. Your feedback means a lot to me and helps me improve as a writer.

Please don't hesitate to reach out to me through

lorenepeachey@gmail.com

I look forward to connecting with my readers and appreciate your support in this literary journey. Your thoughts and comments are valuable to me.

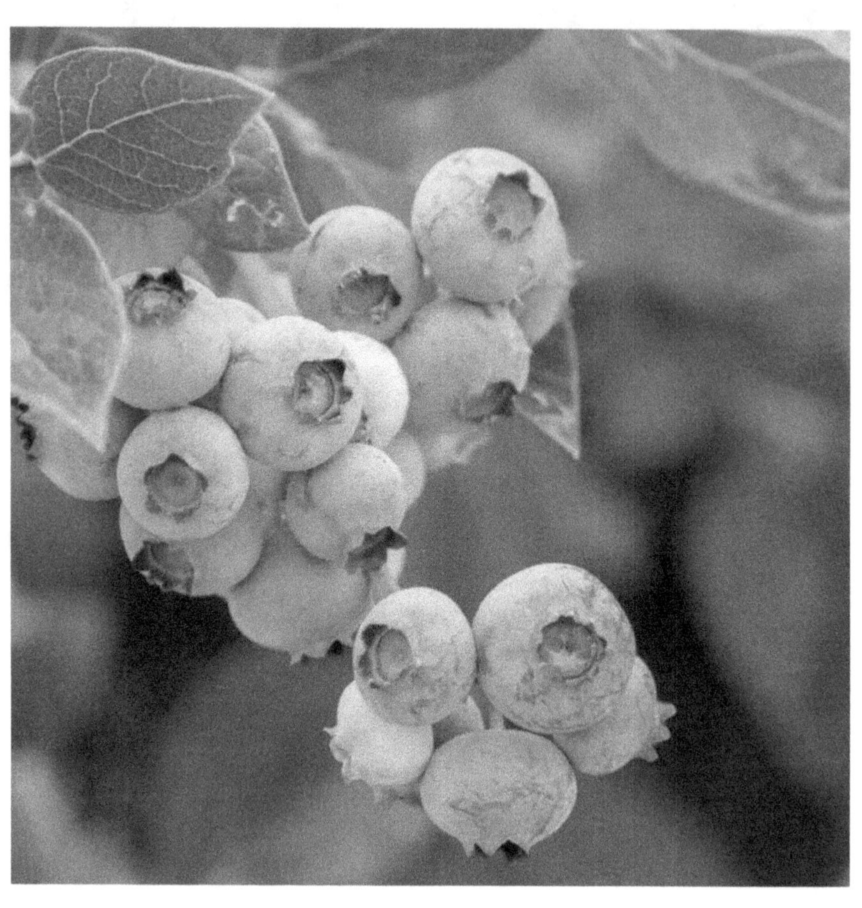

CHAPTER 1

UNDERSTANDING THE

IMPORTANCE OF LOW SUGAR

FOODS

In today's fast-paced and often sedentary lifestyle, the prevalence of high sugar intake has become a major health concern. Excessive sugar consumption is linked to various health issues, including obesity, type 2 diabetes, cardiovascular diseases, and dental problems. Recognizing the importance of low sugar foods and adopting a low sugar diet can significantly contribute to overall well-being.

Benefits of Adopting a Low Sugar Diet:

1. **Weight Management:** High sugar intake is closely associated with weight gain and obesity. Sugar-rich foods tend to be high in empty calories, providing little to no nutritional value. By opting for a low sugar diet, individuals can better regulate their calorie intake, making weight management more achievable.

2. **Blood Sugar Control:** Consuming excess sugar can lead to spikes and crashes in blood sugar levels, contributing to insulin resistance and an increased risk of type 2 diabetes. A low sugar diet helps stabilize blood sugar levels, reducing the likelihood of developing insulin-related disorders.

3. **Heart Health:** Diets high in added sugars are known to elevate triglyceride levels and increase the risk of heart disease. By choosing low sugar alternatives, individuals can support heart health and reduce the risk of cardiovascular complications.

4. **Energy Levels and Mental Clarity:** While sugary foods may provide a quick energy boost, they often lead to energy crashes shortly afterward. Low sugar diets emphasize complex carbohydrates and nutrient-dense foods, providing sustained energy levels and promoting better mental clarity throughout the day.

5. **Reduced Inflammation:** Excessive sugar intake has been linked to chronic inflammation, which is a contributing factor to various diseases, including arthritis and certain cancers. Adopting a low sugar diet can help mitigate inflammation, supporting overall health.

6. **Dental Health:** Sugars contribute to tooth decay by providing a food source for harmful bacteria in the mouth. Choosing low sugar options and practicing good oral hygiene can significantly reduce the risk of dental issues and maintain a healthy smile.

7. **Improved Skin Health:** High sugar consumption has been associated with skin conditions such as acne and premature aging. A low sugar diet, rich in antioxidants and essential nutrients, can promote healthier skin by reducing inflammation and supporting collagen production.

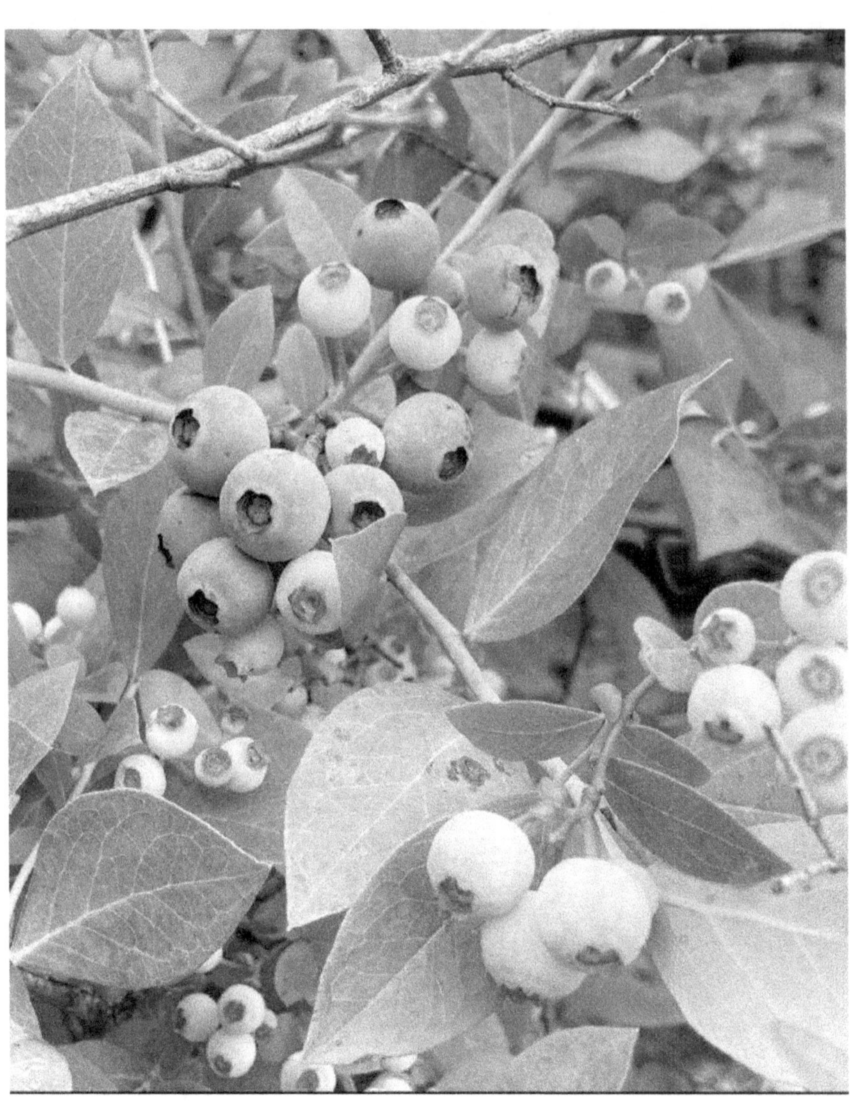

CHAPTER 2

BASICS OF LOW SUGAR EATING

Embracing a low sugar eating approach is a fundamental step toward achieving and maintaining a healthy lifestyle. Understanding the basics of sugar, its variants, recommended daily intake, and how to read nutrition labels can empower individuals to make informed choices about their dietary habits.

Defining Sugar and its Variants:

Sugar is a type of carbohydrate that provides energy to the body. The most common forms of sugar include sucrose (table sugar), fructose (found in fruits), and glucose (a component of carbohydrates). However, it's essential to recognize that sugar comes in various forms, and food labels may use different names to indicate its presence. Some common sugar variants include high fructose corn syrup (HFCS), agave nectar, maltose, and dextrose.

Recommended Daily Sugar Intake:

The World Health Organization (WHO) recommends limiting the intake of added sugars to less than 10% of total daily energy intake. For additional health benefits, a further reduction to below 5% is advised. This equates to roughly 25 grams (6 teaspoons) of added sugar for women and 38 grams (9 teaspoons) for men per day. It's important to note that these guidelines pertain to added sugars and not naturally occurring sugars found in whole foods like fruits and vegetables.

Reading Nutrition Labels Effectively:

1. **Check the Total Sugar Content:** Look at the "Total Sugars" listed on the nutrition label. This includes both natural and added sugars. Be cautious of products with high total sugar content, especially if they are not naturally sweetened.

2. **Identify Added Sugars:** Nutrition labels now include a specific line for "Added Sugars." This distinction helps you differentiate between sugars naturally present in foods and those incorporated during processing. Choose products with lower added sugar content.

3. **Understand Sugar Synonyms:** Sugar can go by many names on ingredient lists. Be on the lookout for terms like sucrose, glucose, fructose, high fructose corn syrup, and other sugar aliases. The closer these ingredients are to the beginning of the list, the higher the sugar content in the product.

4. **Consider Serving Sizes:** Pay attention to serving sizes on the nutrition label. The amount of sugar listed is often based on a single serving, and a product may contain multiple servings. Calculate the total sugar intake accordingly.

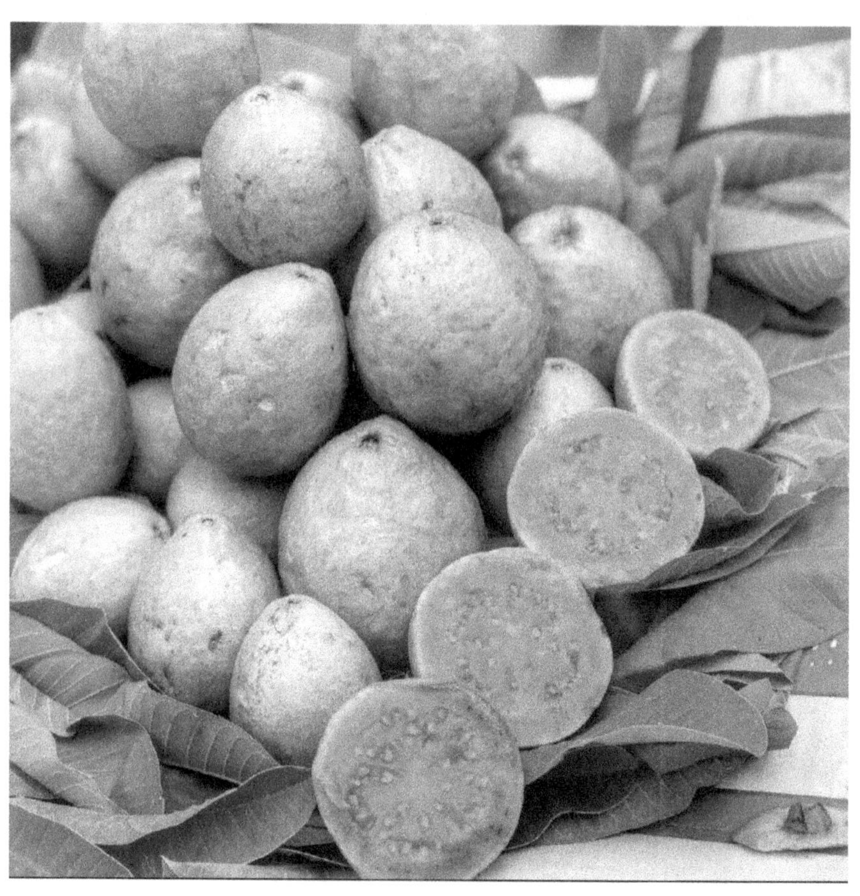

CHAPTER 3

THE IMPACT OF EXCESS SUGAR ON HEALTH

Excessive sugar consumption has emerged as a significant health concern, contributing to various adverse effects on the human body. Understanding the impact of excess sugar on health is crucial for individuals seeking to make informed dietary choices and prioritize their overall well-being.

Obesity and Weight Management:

High sugar intake is strongly linked to obesity. Sugary foods and beverages are often rich in calories and low in nutritional value, leading to overconsumption of empty calories. Additionally, sugar can interfere with the body's natural appetite regulation, promoting a cycle of increased calorie intake. The resulting weight gain not only poses aesthetic concerns but also elevates the risk of developing obesity-related health issues.

Dental Health:

Sugar serves as a fuel source for bacteria in the mouth, contributing to the formation of plaque and causing tooth decay. Frequent consumption of sugary snacks and beverages can erode tooth enamel, leading to cavities and other dental problems. Maintaining good oral hygiene and minimizing sugar intake are essential for preserving dental health and preventing oral issues.

Type 2 Diabetes:

The association between excess sugar consumption and the development of type 2 diabetes is well-established. High sugar intake can lead to insulin resistance, where the body's cells become less responsive to insulin. This, in turn, impairs the regulation of blood sugar levels. Over time, persistent elevated blood sugar levels can contribute to the onset of type 2 diabetes. Adopting a low sugar diet is a key preventive measure in managing diabetes risk.

Cardiovascular Health:

Diets high in added sugars are linked to an increased risk of cardiovascular diseases. Excessive sugar intake is associated with elevated blood pressure, inflammation, and unfavorable lipid profiles. These factors contribute to the development of heart conditions such as hypertension and atherosclerosis. By reducing sugar intake, individuals can positively impact their cardiovascular health and reduce the risk of heart-related complications.

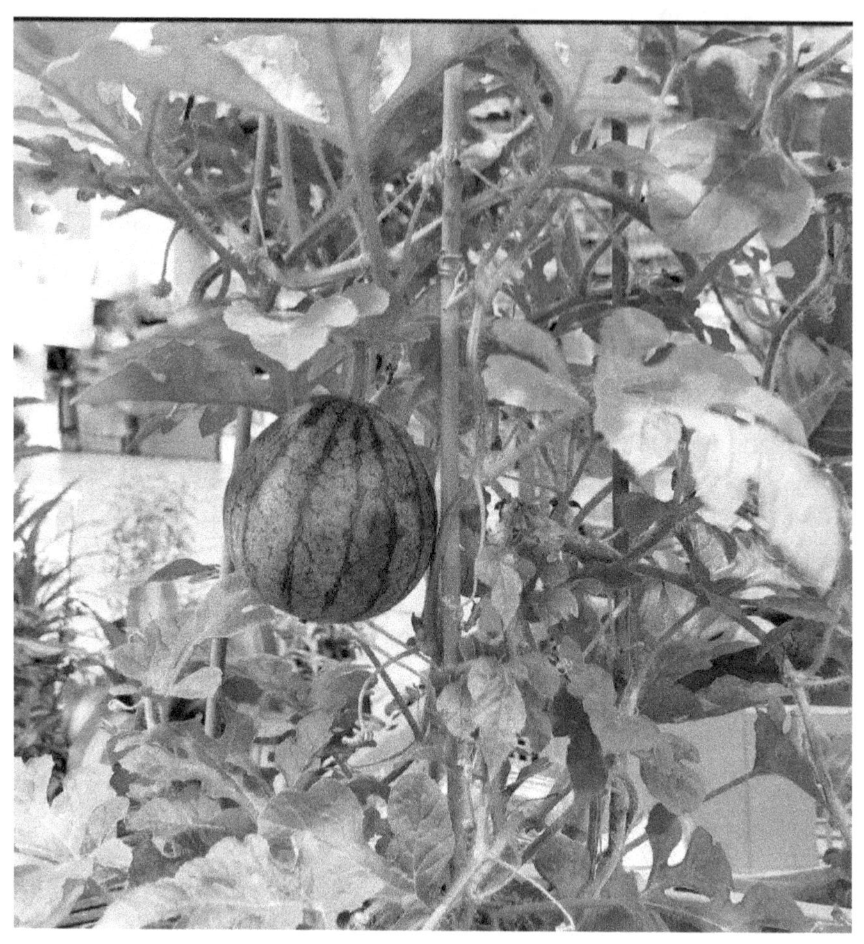

CHAPTER 4

LOW-SUGAR FRUITS

1. **Avocado:**

    - Nutritional Information (per 100g):

        - Calories: 160

        - Total Carbohydrates: 8.53g

        - Dietary Fiber: 6.7g

        - Sugars: 0.66g

        - Healthy Fats: 14.66g

2. **Berries (e.g., Strawberries, Blueberries, Raspberries):**

    - Nutritional Information (per 100g):

        - Calories: 32-57 (depending on the berry)

        - Total Carbohydrates: 5.5-14.5g

        - Dietary Fiber: 2-9g

        - Sugars: 2-7g

        - Rich in Antioxidants and Vitamins

3. **Lemons:**

- Nutritional Information (per 100g):

    - Calories: 29

    - Total Carbohydrates: 9.32g

    - Dietary Fiber: 2.8g

    - Sugars: 2.5g

    - High in Vitamin C

4. **Watermelon:**

- Nutritional Information (per 100g):

    - Calories: 30

    - Total Carbohydrates: 8g

    - Dietary Fiber: 0.4g

    - Sugars: 6.2g

    - Hydrating and a Source of Lycopene

5. **Peaches:**

- Nutritional Information (per 100g):

    - Calories: 39

    - Total Carbohydrates: 9.5g

    - Dietary Fiber: 1.5g

    - Sugars: 8.4g

    - Rich in Vitamins A and C

6. **Cantaloupe:**

- Nutritional Information (per 100g):

    - Calories: 34

    - Total Carbohydrates: 8.2g

    - Dietary Fiber: 0.9g

    - Sugars: 8.2g

    - Excellent Source of Vitamin A

7. **Guava:**

- Nutritional Information (per 100g):

    - Calories: 68

    - Total Carbohydrates: 14g

    - Dietary Fiber: 5.4g

    - Sugars: 9g

    - High in Dietary Fiber and Vitamin C

8. **Kiwi:**

- Nutritional Information (per 100g):

    - Calories: 61

    - Total Carbohydrates: 14.6g

    - Dietary Fiber: 3g

    - Sugars: 9g

    - Rich in Vitamin C and K

9. **Rhubarb:**

- Nutritional Information (per 100g):

    - Calories: 21

    - Total Carbohydrates: 4.5g

    - Dietary Fiber: 1.8g

    - Sugars: 1.1g

    - Low in Calories and Sugars

10. **Papaya:**

- Nutritional Information (per 100g):

    - Calories: 43

    - Total Carbohydrates: 11g

    - Dietary Fiber: 1.7g

    - Sugars: 7g

    - Rich in Vitamin C and A

11. **Blackberries:**

- Nutritional Information (per 100g):

    - Calories: 43

    - Total Carbohydrates: 9.7g

    - Dietary Fiber: 5.3g

    - Sugars: 4.5g

    - Rich in Antioxidants and Vitamin C

CHAPTER 5

LOW-SUGAR VEGETABLES

1. **Broccoli:**

   - Calories: 55

   - Total Carbohydrates: 11.2g

   - Dietary Fiber: 5.1g

   - Sugars: 1.7g

   - Rich in Vitamin C, K, and Folate

2. **Cauliflower:**

   - Calories: 25

   - Total Carbohydrates: 5.3g

   - Dietary Fiber: 2.5g

   - Sugars: 1.9g

   - High in Vitamin C and a Good Source of Fiber

3. **Spinach:**

- Calories: 23

- Total Carbohydrates: 3.6g

- Dietary Fiber: 2.2g

- Sugars: 0.4g

- Packed with Iron, Vitamin A, and Folate

4. **Zucchini:**

- Calories: 17

- Total Carbohydrates: 3.1g

- Dietary Fiber: 1g

- Sugars: 2.1g

- Contains Vitamin C, B6, and Manganese

5. **Asparagus:**

- Calories: 20

- Total Carbohydrates: 3.7g

- Dietary Fiber: 2.1g

- Sugars: 1.9g

- High in Folate, Vitamin K, and Antioxidants

6. **Cabbage:**

- Calories: 25

- Total Carbohydrates: 5.8g

- Dietary Fiber: 2.5g

- Sugars: 3.2g

- Rich in Vitamin C and K

7. **Bell Peppers (Green):**

- Calories: 20

- Total Carbohydrates: 4.6g

- Dietary Fiber: 1.7g

- Sugars: 2.9g

- Excellent Source of Vitamin C

8. **Mushrooms:**

- Calories: 22

- Total Carbohydrates: 3.3g

- Dietary Fiber: 1g

- Sugars: 1.7g

- Good Source of B Vitamins and Selenium

9. **Cucumbers:**

- Calories: 16

- Total Carbohydrates: 3.6g

- Dietary Fiber: 0.5g

- Sugars: 1.8g

- Hydrating and Contains Vitamin K

10. **Brussels Sprouts:**

- Calories: 43

- Total Carbohydrates: 9g

- Dietary Fiber: 3.8g

- Sugars: 2.2g

- High in Vitamin C and K

11. **Kale:**

- Calories: 50

- Total Carbohydrates: 10g

- Dietary Fiber: 2g

- Sugars: 0.9g

- Rich in Vitamin A, C, and K

CHAPTER 6

LEAN PROTEINS

1. **Chicken Breast (Grilled):**

   - Calories: 165

   - Protein: 31g

   - Total Fat: 3.6g

   - Saturated Fat: 1g

   - Carbohydrates: 0g

2. **Turkey Breast (Roasted):**

   - Calories: 135

   - Protein: 30g

   - Total Fat: 1g

   - Saturated Fat: 0.3g

   - Carbohydrates: 0g

3. **Fish (Cod, Baked):**

- Calories: 105

- Protein: 23g

- Total Fat: 1g

- Saturated Fat: 0.2g

- Carbohydrates: 0g

4. **Salmon (Baked):**

- Calories: 206

- Protein: 22g

- Total Fat: 13g

- Saturated Fat: 2g

- Carbohydrates: 0g

5. **Egg Whites (Boiled):**

- Calories: 52

- Protein: 11g

- Total Fat: 0.2g

- Saturated Fat: 0g

- Carbohydrates: 0.6g

6. **Lean Ground Beef (90% lean):**

   - Calories: 250

   - Protein: 26g

   - Total Fat: 17g

   - Saturated Fat: 7g

   - Carbohydrates: 0g

7. **Tofu (Firm):**

   - Calories: 144

   - Protein: 15g

   - Total Fat: 8g

   - Saturated Fat: 1.2g

   - Carbohydrates: 3.9g

8. **Greek Yogurt (Plain, Non-fat):**

   - Calories: 59

   - Protein: 10g

   - Total Fat: 0.4g

   - Saturated Fat: 0.2g

   - Carbohydrates: 3.6g

9. **Shrimp (Boiled):**

- Calories: 99

- Protein: 24g

- Total Fat: 0.3g

- Saturated Fat: 0.1g

- Carbohydrates: 0g

10. **Skinless Turkey Sausage (Grilled):**

- Calories: 153

- Protein: 16g

- Total Fat: 9g

- Saturated Fat: 2.7g

- Carbohydrates: 1.4g

11. **Cottage Cheese (Low-fat):**

- Calories: 72

- Protein: 12g

- Total Fat: 1.2g

- Saturated Fat: 0.7g

- Carbohydrates: 3.3g

CHAPTER 7

WHOLE GRAINS

1. **Quinoa (Cooked):**

   - Calories: 120

   - Total Carbohydrates: 21g

   - Dietary Fiber: 2.8g

   - Sugars: 0.9g

   - Protein: 4.1g

2. **Brown Rice (Cooked):**

   - Calories: 111

   - Total Carbohydrates: 23g

   - Dietary Fiber: 1.8g

   - Sugars: 0.4g

   - Protein: 2.6g

3. **Oats (Rolled, Cooked):**

- Calories: 71

- Total Carbohydrates: 12g

- Dietary Fiber: 1.7g

- Sugars: 0.2g

- Protein: 2.5g

4. **Barley (Cooked):**

- Calories: 123

- Total Carbohydrates: 28g

- Dietary Fiber: 3g

- Sugars: 0.4g

- Protein: 2.3g

5. **Buckwheat (Cooked):**

- Calories: 92

- Total Carbohydrates: 19g

- Dietary Fiber: 2.7g

- Sugars: 0.3g

- Protein: 3.4g

6. **Whole Wheat Pasta (Cooked):**

- Calories: 124

- Total Carbohydrates: 25g

- Dietary Fiber: 4g

- Sugars: 0.5g

- Protein: 5g

7. **Farro (Cooked):**

- Calories: 170

- Total Carbohydrates: 35g

- Dietary Fiber: 5.3g

- Sugars: 0.4g

- Protein: 6.5g

8. **Millet (Cooked):**

- Calories: 119

- Total Carbohydrates: 23g

- Dietary Fiber: 1.3g

- Sugars: 0.1g

- Protein: 3.5g

9. **Quinoa Flakes (Cooked):**

- Calories: 60

- Total Carbohydrates: 12g

- Dietary Fiber: 1.5g

- Sugars: 0.1g

- Protein: 1.9g

10. **Wild Rice (Cooked):**

- Calories: 101

- Total Carbohydrates: 21g

- Dietary Fiber: 1.8g

- Sugars: 0.3g

- Protein: 3.9g

11. **Spelt (Cooked):**

- Calories: 135

- Total Carbohydrates: 28g

- Dietary Fiber: 3.7g

- Sugars: 0.4g

- Protein: 5.3g

CHAPTER 8

DAIRY AND DAIRY

ALTERNATIVES

1. **Greek Yogurt (Plain, Non-fat):**

   - Calories: 59

   - Protein: 10g

   - Total Fat: 0.4g

   - Saturated Fat: 0.2g

   - Sugars: 3.6g

2. **Skim Milk:**

   - Calories: 34

   - Protein: 3.4g

   - Total Fat: 0.2g

   - Saturated Fat: 0.1g

   - Sugars: 4.8g

3. **Cottage Cheese (Low-fat):**

- Calories: 72

- Protein: 12g

- Total Fat: 1.2g

- Saturated Fat: 0.7g

- Sugars: 3.3g

4. **Almond Milk (Unsweetened):**

- Calories: 13

- Protein: 0.5g

- Total Fat: 1.1g

- Saturated Fat: 0.1g

- Sugars: 0g

5. **Coconut Yogurt (Unsweetened):**

- Calories: 22

- Protein: 0.5g

- Total Fat: 1.9g

- Saturated Fat: 1.7g

- Sugars: 0.6g

6. **Feta Cheese (Reduced Fat):**

- Calories: 134

- Protein: 16g

- Total Fat: 6.2g

- Saturated Fat: 4.1g

- Sugars: 0.4g

7. **Soy Milk (Unsweetened):**

- Calories: 33

- Protein: 3.3g

- Total Fat: 1.7g

- Saturated Fat: 0.2g

- Sugars: 0.3g

8. **Ricotta Cheese (Part-skim):**

- Calories: 174

- Protein: 14g

- Total Fat: 10g

- Saturated Fat: 6.4g

- Sugars: 0.6g

9. **Plain Yogurt (Whole Milk):**

- Calories: 61

- Protein: 3.5g

- Total Fat: 3.3g

- Saturated Fat: 2.1g

- Sugars: 3.6g

10. **Cashew Milk (Unsweetened):**

- Calories: 13

- Protein: 0.5g

- Total Fat: 1g

- Saturated Fat: 0.2g

- Sugars: 0g

11. **Mozzarella Cheese (Part-skim):**

- Calories: 300

- Protein: 25g

- Total Fat: 21g

- Saturated Fat: 13g

- Sugars: 1g

CHAPTER 9

HIGH-SUGAR FOODS

1. **Regular Soda (Cola):**

    - Calories: 42

    - Total Carbohydrates: 10.6g

    - Sugars: 10.6g

2. **Candy (Hard Candy, Various Types):**

    - Calories: 394

    - Total Carbohydrates: 98g

    - Sugars: 63g

3. **Milk Chocolate:**

    - Calories: 546

    - Total Carbohydrates: 59g

    - Sugars: 51g

4. **Fruit Juice (Orange Juice, Unsweetened):**

- Calories: 45

- Total Carbohydrates: 8.2g

- Sugars: 8.2g

5. **Flavored Yogurt (Fruit Flavored, Sweetened):**

- Calories: 87

- Total Carbohydrates: 14.5g

- Sugars: 12.4g

6. **Cakes and Pastries (Various Types):**

- Calories: 412

- Total Carbohydrates: 57g

- Sugars: 38g

7. **Sweetened Breakfast Cereal:**

- Calories: 375

- Total Carbohydrates: 88g

- Sugars: 40g

8. **Energy Drinks:**

- Calories: 45

- Total Carbohydrates: 11g

- Sugars: 10g

9. **Commercially Prepared Ice Cream:**

- Calories: 207

- Total Carbohydrates: 26g

- Sugars: 24g

10. **Granola Bars (Sweetened):**

- Calories: 466

- Total Carbohydrates: 69g

- Sugars: 34g

11. **Honey:**

- Calories: 304

- Total Carbohydrates: 82g

- Sugars: 82g

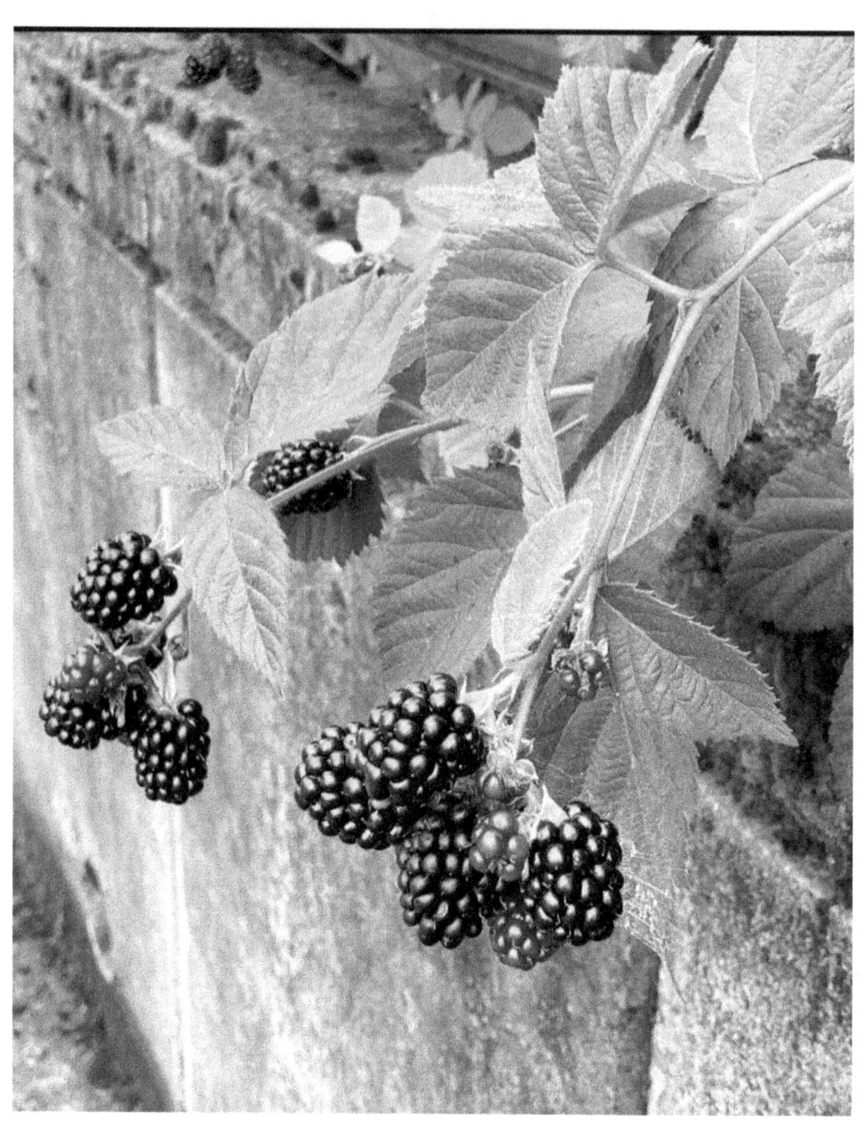

CONCLUSION

As we come to the final pages of this culinary odyssey, I am filled with gratitude and a deep sense of fulfillment. This journey has been more than just a compilation of recipes; it's been a shared exploration of the transformative power of low-sugar living. From the depths of my heart, I thank you for allowing me to be a part of your quest for a healthier, more vibrant life.

As you've ventured through the chapters, I hope you've found not just a collection of dishes but a roadmap to a new way of nourishing your body and soul. The essence of this book is not confined to its pages; it extends into your kitchens, your dining tables, and the very fabric of your daily lives. I believe in the profound impact of mindful eating, and I hope that belief resonates with you as well.

Remember, this is not a journey with a fixed destination; it's an ongoing exploration with infinite possibilities. As you experiment with these recipes, I encourage you to make them your own. Tailor them to suit your tastes, preferences, and dietary needs. The magic lies not just in the ingredients but in the personal touch you bring to each dish.

Your feedback is a cherished gift – a dialogue that continues long after you've closed the book. I am eager to hear about your experiences, the moments of joy in your kitchen, and the victories in your journey toward a healthier lifestyle. Let this book be a starting point for conversations about wellness, about embracing a life where food is not just sustenance but a source of joy and vitality.

Please share your thoughts, your challenges, and your triumphs. Your feedback fuels the fire of inspiration, and it's a reminder that we are all on this journey together. Whether you've experienced a breakthrough in your well-being or faced hurdles in adopting a low-sugar lifestyle, your insights are invaluable.

In closing, I want to express my heartfelt wish that this book becomes a companion in your ongoing pursuit of health and happiness. May it inspire you to savor each moment, each bite, and each day with a newfound appreciation for the incredible vessel that is your body.

Thank you for entrusting me with a small part of your journey. As you embark on the adventure that lies ahead, may your life be filled with the richness of flavors, the nourishment of wholesome ingredients, and the joy that comes from taking charge of your well-being.

Here's to a life well-lived, to the joy of mindful eating, and to the vibrant tapestry of flavors that awaits you. Until we meet again, happy cooking and even happier living!

BONUS CHAPTER 1

LOW-SUGAR RECIPES

Grilled Lemon Herb Chicken

Cooking Time: 20 minutes

Servings: 4

Ingredients:

- 4 boneless, skinless chicken breasts

- 2 tablespoons olive oil

- Juice of 2 lemons

- 2 cloves garlic, minced

- 1 teaspoon dried oregano

- Salt and pepper to taste

Instructions:

1. Preheat grill to medium-high heat.

2. In a bowl, mix olive oil, lemon juice, minced garlic, oregano, salt, and pepper.

3. Marinate chicken breasts in the mixture for 15 minutes.

4. Grill chicken for about 7-8 minutes per side or until fully cooked.

5. Serve with your favorite low-sugar vegetables.

Nutritional Information: Approx. 250 calories, 30g protein, 12g fat, 3g carbs

Quinoa Salad with Vegetables

Cooking Time: 15 minutes

Servings: 4

Ingredients:

- 1 cup quinoa, cooked

- 1 cup cherry tomatoes, halved

- 1 cucumber, diced

- 1 bell pepper, chopped

- 1/4 cup feta cheese, crumbled

- Fresh basil leaves

Instructions:

1. In a large bowl, combine cooked quinoa, cherry tomatoes, cucumber, bell pepper, and feta cheese.

2. Add fresh basil leaves.

3. Drizzle with olive oil and balsamic vinegar, and season with salt and pepper.

4. Toss gently and serve chilled.

Nutritional Information: Approx. 220 calories, 7g protein, 8g fat, 30g carbs

Baked Salmon with Lemon and Dill

Cooking Time: 25 minutes

Servings: 2

Ingredients:

- 2 salmon fillets

- 1 lemon, thinly sliced

- Fresh dill

- Salt and pepper to taste

Instructions:

1. Preheat oven to 375°F (190°C).

2. Place salmon fillets on a baking sheet lined with parchment paper.

3. Season with salt and pepper, top with lemon slices, and sprinkle fresh dill.

4. Bake for 20-25 minutes or until salmon flakes easily with a fork.

5. Serve with steamed vegetables or a side salad.

Nutritional Information: Approx. 300 calories, 25g protein, 15g fat, 5g carbs

Avocado and Tomato Salad

Cooking Time: 10 minutes

Servings: 2

Ingredients:

- 2 avocados, diced

- 1 cup cherry tomatoes, halved

- Red onion, thinly sliced

- Fresh cilantro, chopped

- Lime juice, salt, and pepper to taste

Instructions:

1. In a bowl, combine diced avocados, cherry tomatoes, red onion, and cilantro.

2. Drizzle with lime juice and season with salt and pepper.

3. Toss gently and serve immediately.

Nutritional Information: Approx. 180 calories, 2g protein, 15g fat, 12g carbs

Chicken and Vegetable Stir-Fry

Cooking Time: 15 minutes

Servings: 4

Ingredients:

- 1 lb boneless, skinless chicken breast, sliced

- 2 cups broccoli florets

- 1 red bell pepper, sliced

- 1 carrot, julienned

- 2 tablespoons soy sauce

- 1 tablespoon sesame oil

- 1 teaspoon ginger, minced

- 2 cloves garlic, minced

Instructions:

1. In a wok or skillet, heat sesame oil over medium-high heat.

2. Add sliced chicken and cook until browned.

3. Add broccoli, bell pepper, carrot, ginger, and garlic.

4. Stir in soy sauce and cook until vegetables are tender.

5. Serve over cauliflower rice.

Nutritional Information: Approx. 280 calories, 30g protein, 8g fat, 18g carbs

Spinach and Feta Stuffed Chicken Breast

Cooking Time: 30 minutes

Servings: 4

Ingredients:

- 4 boneless, skinless chicken breasts

- 2 cups fresh spinach

- 1/2 cup feta cheese, crumbled

- 2 tablespoons olive oil

- Garlic powder, salt, and pepper to taste

Instructions:

1. Preheat oven to 375°F (190°C).

2. In a skillet, sauté spinach with olive oil until wilted.

3. Butterfly each chicken breast and stuff with spinach and feta.

4. Season with garlic powder, salt, and pepper.

5. Bake for 25-30 minutes or until chicken is cooked through.

Nutritional Information: Approx. 230 calories, 30g protein, 10g fat, 4g carbs

Cauliflower and Broccoli Soup

Cooking Time: 25 minutes

Servings: 6

Ingredients:

- 1 head cauliflower, chopped
- 2 cups broccoli florets
- 1 onion, diced
- 2 cloves garlic, minced
- 4 cups vegetable broth
- 1 cup unsweetened almond milk
- Fresh parsley for garnish

Instructions:

1. In a large pot, sauté onions and garlic until softened.

2. Add cauliflower, broccoli, and vegetable broth. Bring to a boil.

3. Reduce heat and simmer until vegetables are tender.

4. Use an immersion blender to puree the soup.

5. Stir in almond milk, season with salt and pepper, and garnish with fresh parsley.

Nutritional Information: Approx. 120 calories, 4g protein, 5g fat, 16g carbs

Shrimp and Avocado Lettuce Wraps

Cooking Time: 15 minutes

Servings: 4

Ingredients:

- 1 lb shrimp, peeled and deveined

- 2 avocados, diced

- 1 cup cherry tomatoes, halved

- Butter lettuce leaves

- Lime juice, cilantro, salt, and pepper to taste

Instructions:

1. Cook shrimp in a skillet until pink and opaque.

2. In a bowl, combine shrimp, diced avocados, and cherry tomatoes.

3. Drizzle with lime juice, sprinkle with cilantro, and season with salt and pepper.

4. Spoon the mixture into lettuce leaves and serve.

Nutritional Information: Approx. 220 calories, 25g protein, 10g fat, 8g carbs

Zucchini Noodles with Pesto

Cooking Time: 15 minutes

Servings: 2

Ingredients:

- 2 large zucchinis, spiralized
- 1/2 cup cherry tomatoes, halved
- 1/4 cup pine nuts
- 1/2 cup fresh basil leaves
- 1/4 cup Parmesan cheese, grated
- 2 cloves garlic
- 1/4 cup olive oil

Instructions:

1. In a blender, combine basil, pine nuts, Parmesan, garlic, and olive oil. Blend until smooth.

2. Spiralize zucchinis into noodles.

3. Toss zucchini noodles with cherry tomatoes and pesto.

4. Season with salt and pepper, and serve.

Nutritional Information: Approx. 220 calories, 5g protein, 18g fat, 8g carbs

Berry Chia Seed Pudding

Preparation Time: 5 minutes

Chilling Time: 4 hours

Servings: 2

Ingredients:

- 1 cup unsweetened almond milk

- 1/4 cup chia seeds

- 1 tablespoon honey or maple syrup

- 1/2 teaspoon vanilla extract

- Mixed berries for topping

Instructions:

1. In a jar, mix almond milk, chia seeds, honey, and vanilla extract.

2. Stir well and refrigerate for at least 4 hours or overnight.

3. Before serving, top with mixed berries.

Nutritional Information: Approx. 180 calories, 4g protein, 10g fat, 20g carbs

IF YOU WANT MORE RECIPES, YOU CAN CHECK OUT OTHER BOOKS BY THE AUTHOR

LOW POTASSIUM DIET COOKBOOK FOR SENIORS

KIDNEY DISEASE DIET COOKBOOK FOR WOMEN

LOW SODIUM COOKBOOK FOR CONGESTIVE HEART FAILURE

TYPE 2 DIABETES COOKBOOK FOR SENIORS

GLUTEN-FREE AIR FRYER COOKBOOK

TO GET ACCESS TO MORE BOOKS BY THE AUTHOR SCAN THE QR CODE

BONUS CHAPTER 2

21 DAY MEAL PLAN

Day	Breakfast	Lunch	Dinner
1	Avocado Toast	Quinoa Salad with Vegetables	Grilled Lemon Herb Chicken with Broccoli
2	Greek Yogurt Parfait	Spinach and Feta Stuffed Chicken Breast	Cauliflower and Broccoli Soup
3	Berry Chia Seed Pudding	Shrimp and Avocado Lettuce Wraps	Baked Salmon with Lemon and Dill
4	Oatmeal with Berries	Chicken and Vegetable Stir-Fry	Zucchini Noodles with Pesto
5	Scrambled Eggs with Spinach	Cottage Cheese and Tomato Salad	Quinoa Salad with Vegetables

6	Almond Butter Smoothie	Turkey Lettuce Wraps	Chicken and Vegetable Stir-Fry
7	Whole Grain Toast with Peanut Butter	Avocado and Tomato Salad	Grilled Lemon Herb Chicken with Broccoli
8	Vegetable Omelette	Chickpea Salad	Baked Salmon with Lemon and Dill
9	Greek Yogurt with Berries	Zucchini Noodles with Pesto	Spinach and Feta Stuffed Chicken Breast
10	Cottage Cheese Pancakes	Quinoa Salad with Vegetables	Shrimp and Avocado Lettuce Wraps
11	Smoothie Bowl	Chicken and Vegetable Stir-Fry	Cauliflower and Broccoli Soup
12	Chia Seed Pudding with Almond Milk	Avocado Toast	Baked Salmon with Lemon and Dill

13	Scrambled Tofu with Vegetables	Turkey Lettuce Wraps	Grilled Lemon Herb Chicken with Broccoli
14	Whole Grain Waffles	Chickpea Salad	Zucchini Noodles with Pesto
15	Greek Yogurt Parfait	Quinoa Salad with Vegetables	Cauliflower and Broccoli Soup
16	Oatmeal with Nuts and Seeds	Spinach and Feta Stuffed Chicken Breast	Chicken and Vegetable Stir-Fry
17	Almond Butter Smoothie	Cottage Cheese and Tomato Salad	Shrimp and Avocado Lettuce Wraps
18	Avocado Toast	Chickpea Salad	Baked Salmon with Lemon and Dill
19	Berry Chia Seed Pudding	Turkey Lettuce Wraps	Zucchini Noodles with Pesto
20	Greek Yogurt with Berries	Quinoa Salad with Vegetables	Spinach and Feta Stuffed

			Chicken Breast
21	Vegetable Omelette	Shrimp and Avocado Lettuce Wraps	Cauliflower and Broccoli Soup